I Remember Series
Bible Stories

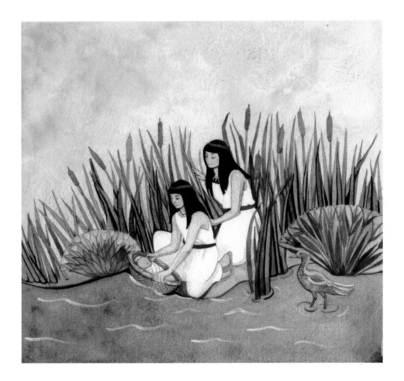

Brenda C. Poulos
Illustrated by Jenny Reynish

Published by Connections Press

Printed in The United States of America

Formatted by Ruth L. Snyder http://ruthlsnyder.com

ISBN-13: 978-1985584150

ISBN-10: 1985584158

First Edition

In loving memory of Randy Pawlicki.

He brought love and laughter to all who knew him.

1942-2017

I Remember

I remember Bible stories
I heard them as I grew.
Truths from God's Holy Word
I'd like to share with you...

Resources to help trigger memories of events and lessons learned in the past are especially important for people experiencing Alzheimer's.

The interactive nature of picture books helps the brain retain neurological connections, prompting individuals to maintain language, focus, and attention span.

Listening to words and looking at pictures, along with touching and turning pages, provides a much-needed multi-sensory experience.

This second book in the *I Remember* series created for individuals with Alzheimer's by Brenda Poulos, *I Remember Bible Stories,* will be sure to spark welcoming memories.

~ Susan A. Kasprak, BSW, Certified Dementia Practioner Director of Sales, Sunrise Assisted Living, Gilbert, Arizona

"For whatsoever things were written aforetime were written for our learning, that we through patience and comfort of the scriptures might have hope."

Romans 15:4

INTRODUCTION

Although short-term memory is commonly lost by millions of people diagnosed with Alzheimer's, they may still retain many of their childhood memories.

Being convinced that these individuals would be comforted by picture books focusing on activities, songs, and stories they enjoyed—and still remember—from their early years, I began to write a series of Interactive Picture Books for Alzheimer's patients.

The first book in the series, *I Remember the Seasons,* focused on seasonal activities these individuals recall enjoying in their childhood—things such as sledding, going on hayrides and playing baseball.

This second book will act as a catalyst for memories of beloved Bible Stories. My amazing illustrator, Jenny Reynish, and I have prayed over each of these pages during the entire creative process, in the hope that this book will be a blessing to yourself and someone you know and love.

The scriptures above each picture, as well as the questions below them, will serve to stimulate memories of each Bible story.

The stories are presented in no particular order.

Brenda Poulos

Benefits of Interactive Picture Books for People with Alzheimer's

1) Aids in language retention.

2) Helps the brain retain neurological connections.

3) Encourages interactive experiences with each story.

4) Prompts the person to maintain focus and attention.

5) Listening to words and looking a pictures, touching and turning pages, provide a multi-sensory experience.

How To Use This Book

This book will stimulate the recall of enjoyable Bible stories for people with Alzheimer's, while connecting them in a meaningful way to their caregivers—whether family members or health care professionals.

- Have the person with Alzheimer's read the text aloud, if he/she would like to and/or is able. If not, it should be read aloud by the caregiver.

- **If you are unfamiliar with these stories,** a synopsis of each one is available at the back of this book. You may want to read these first, to prepare you for the question/discussion activity. Also, instead of just reading the Bible verse on the picture page, feel free to read the entire synopsis aloud to the individual with Alzheimer's, especially those who had difficulty remembering the stories.

- **Poems, and illustrations, are followed by italicized discussion questions.** Please allow time for this activity, for this is the key in forming desired connections and developing relationships. Feel free to substitute, add, or delete questions, as you see appropriate.

- Utilize the questions as a catalyst for meaningful discussions, rather than accepting simple yes/no answers. Talk *with* the person, evoking emotions and helping him/her access past memories as they enjoy forming valuable connections with *you.*

I Remember Bible Stories

I Remember Bible Stories,
Lessons from my youth.
I recall beloved scriptures,
God's Word, I know, is truth.

I Remember Bible Stories,
About the saints of old,
They tell of God's great love,
As salvation's plan unfolds.

I Remember Bible Stories,
And listening once more,
They bring me hope and peace,
Just as they did before.

I Remember Series

Bible Stories

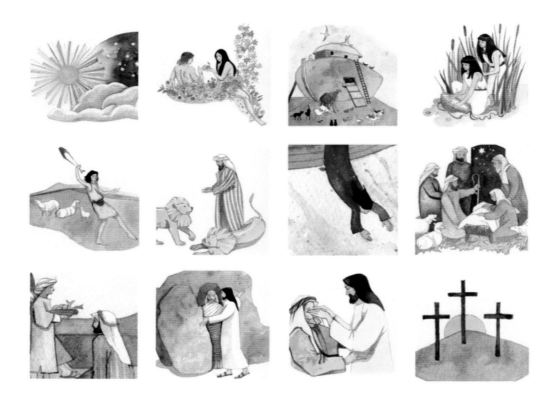

I Remember
THE STORY OF CREATION

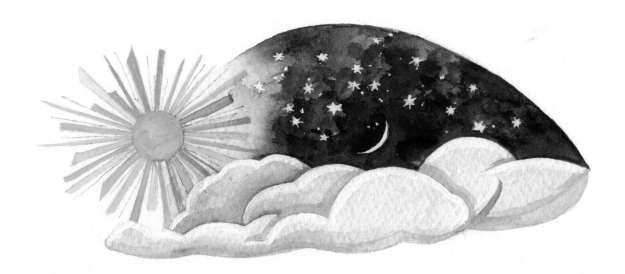

God created the heavens,

The sun, the moon, the stars.

Then mankind, plants, and animals

On this wonderful world of ours.

Genesis 1:1- "In the beginning, God created the heavens and the earth."

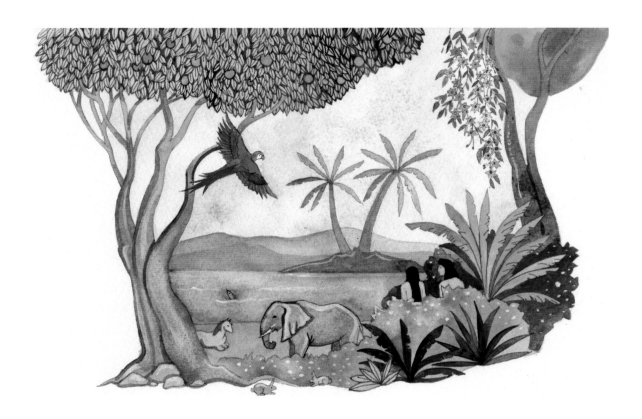

Who created the heavens, the earth, people, and animals? How long did it take? What did he create the first day? The second? The third? The fourth? The fifth? The sixth? What did he do the seventh day?

I Remember

THE STORY OF ADAM AND EVE

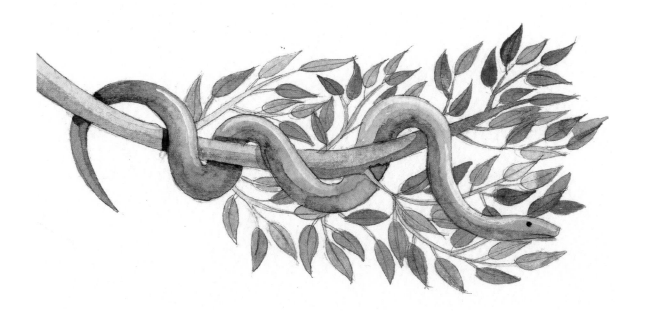

Don't eat the fruit, the Lord God said, or surely you shall die.

Instead they listened to the snake; he deceived them with a lie.

Genesis 2:9- "The Lord God made all kinds of trees grow out of the ground—trees that were pleasing to the eye and good for food. In the middle of the garden were the tree of life and the tree of the knowledge of good and evil."

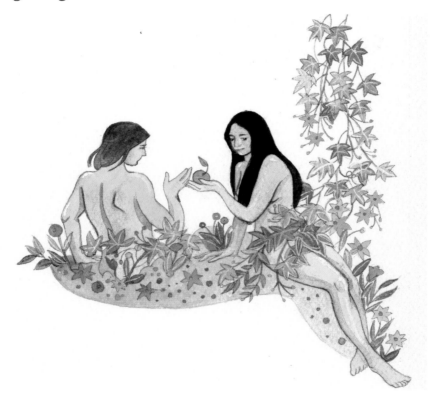

Where did Adam and Eve live? Who lied to them? What lie did he tell them? What happened when Adam and Eve ate fruit from the garden? How did God punish them?

I Remember
THE STORY OF BABY MOSES

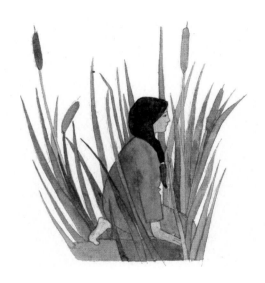

His mother hid the baby

In the river amongst the reeds,

And Pharaoh's daughter saved him

From her father's death decree.

Exodus 2:5,6- "Then Pharaoh's daughter went down to the Nile to bathe, and her attendants were walking along the riverbank. She saw the basket among the reeds and sent her female slave to get it. She opened it and saw the baby. He was crying, and she felt sorry for him. 'This is one of the Hebrew babies,' she said."

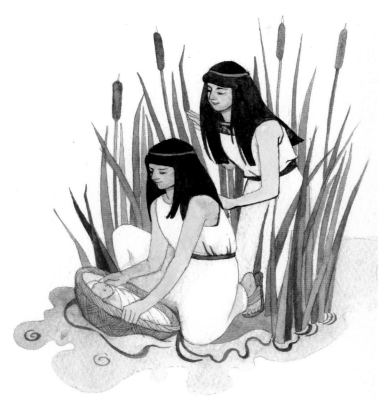

Where did the baby's mother hide him? Who found the baby? What did she name the baby? Once the baby was weaned, where did he go to live?

I Remember

THE STORY OF DAVID AND GOLIATH

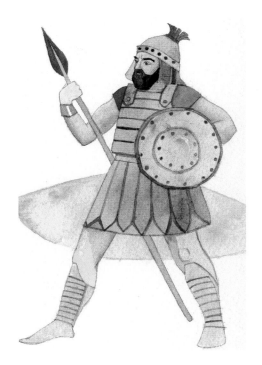

David faced the giant with a slingshot and a stone,

The giant fell, the battle won, and David's faith was shown.

I Samuel 17:48,49 - "As the Philistine moved closer to attack him, David ran quickly toward the battle line to meet him. Reaching into his bag and taking out a stone, he slung it and struck the Philistine on the forehead. The stone sank into his forehead, and he fell facedown on the ground."

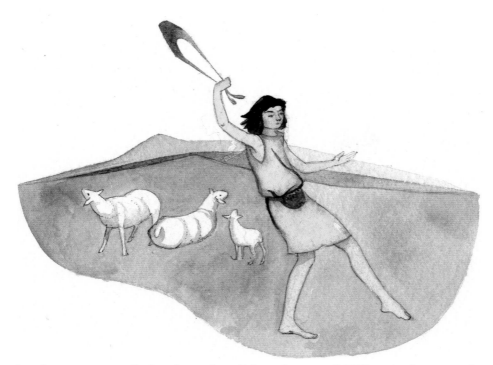

What is the name of the boy in this picture? Why is he on the battlefield? What is the giant's name? What happens to the giant in this story? What does this story teach us about God? Tell about a time when you used what you learned from this story in your own life.

I Remember

THE STORY OF DANIEL AND THE LIONS' DEN

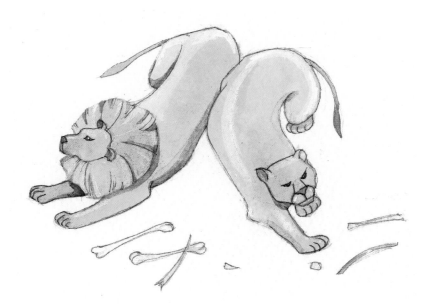

"I'm here," Daniel told the king, "You needn't be alarmed.

God's angel shut the lions' mouths and I was left unharmed!"

Daniel 6: 19b-22a He (the king) called to Daniel in an anguished voice, "Daniel, servant of the living God, has your God whom you serve continually, been able to rescue you from the lions?"

Daniel answered, "May the king live forever! My God sent his angel, and he shut the mouths of the lions."

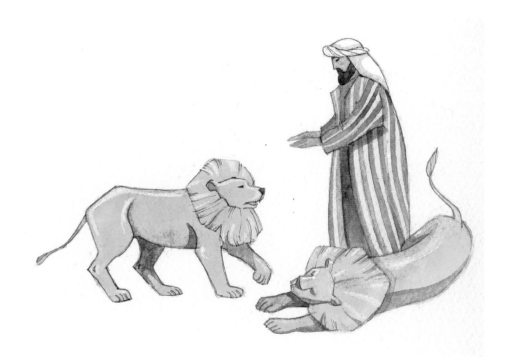

Who did Daniel worship? What law had Daniel broken? What was his punishment? Did the lions harm Daniel? Who kept Daniel safe? Who did Daniel praise?

I Remember

THE STORY OF JONAH AND THE WHALE

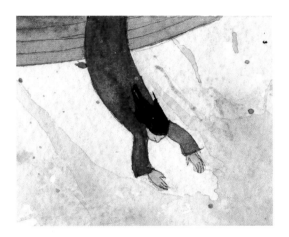

Inside the belly of the whale,

Jonah learned his lesson.

He would no longer flee from God,

But follow His direction.

Jonah 1: 17- "Now the Lord provided a huge fish to swallow Jonah, and Jonah was in the belly of the fish three days and three nights."

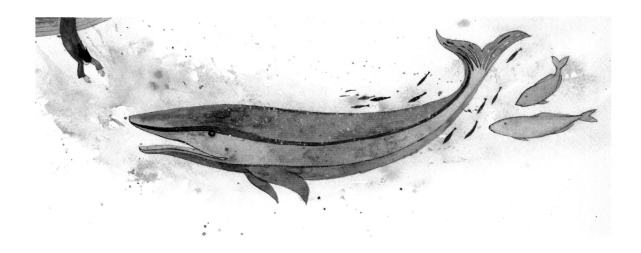

What is the name of the man in this Bible story? What did God tell Jonah to do? What did Jonah do instead? When he refused to obey God, what happened to him? How long was he there? When he was returned to dry land, did he follow God's new command? Why do you suppose he obeyed this time?

I Remember

THE STORY OF NOAH AND THE ARK

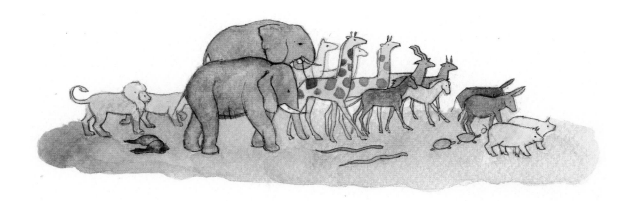

Following Noah, two by two,

The animals entered the ark.

Tigers, cows, and kangaroos,

Even elephants and aardvarks!

Genesis 7: 7-10 "Noah and his sons and his wife and his sons' wives entered the ark to escape the waters of the flood. Pairs of clean and unclean animals, of birds and of all creatures that move along the ground, male and female, came to Noah and entered the ark, as God had commanded Noah. And after seven days the floodwaters came on the earth."

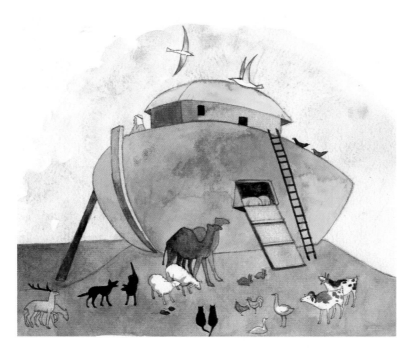

Why did God send the flood to destroy the earth? Name some of the animals that Noah led onto the ark. Why was Noah saved from the floodwaters? Who were the other people that were saved? What sign did God put in the sky as a sign of His promise never to destroy the earth again by a flood?

I Remember

THE STORY OF THE BIRTH OF JESUS

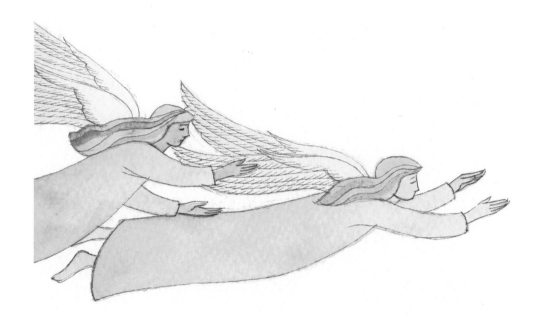

God's plan was perfect,

The Bible tells us so.

He sent Jesus to us,

His infinite love to show.

Luke 2:11,12- "Today in the town of David a Savior has been born to you; he is the Messiah, the Lord. This will be a sign to you: You will find the baby wrapped in cloths and lying in a manger."

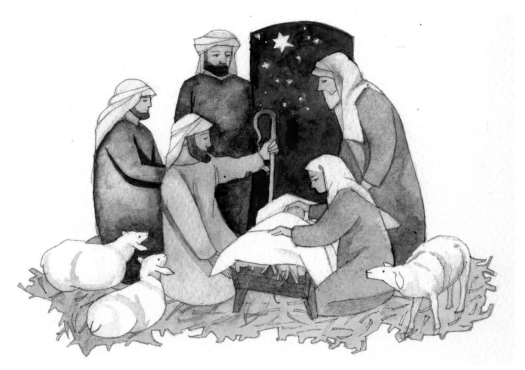

What was the baby's name? Who was his mother? Why were they staying in a stable? What sign did the shepherds and wise men see in the sky? Why was the birth of this baby so special to them? What did they bring to him? Who did this baby grow up to be? What miraculous thing did he do for us?

I Remember

THE STORY OF THE LOAVES AND FISHES

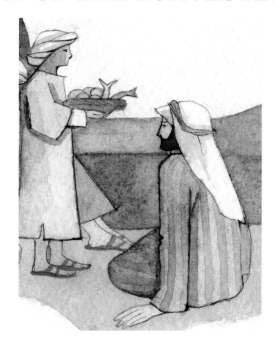

Jesus performed a miracle

As he bowed his head and prayed.

A boy's lunch of loaves and fishes

Fed five thousand men that day.

John 12:13- "So they gathered twelve baskets with the pieces of the five barley loaves left over by those who had eaten."

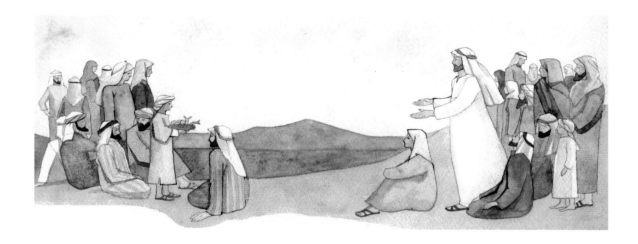

Who did the people want to hear preach? Why? What do you suppose the preaching was about? When the people got hungry, Jesus asked the disciples to feed them. What was the problem? A little boy had brought a lunch with him. What was it? He brought the food to Jesus. What did Jesus do with it? Was it enough to feed the entire crowd? How do you know?

I Remember
THE STORY OF LAZARUS

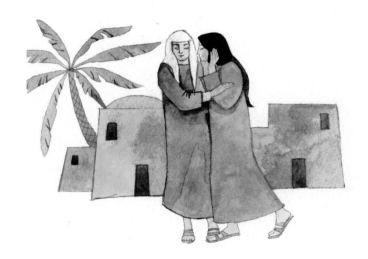

"Lazarus, come forth," were the words Jesus said.

And, with them he raised his dear friend from the dead.

John 11:43b-"Jesus called in a loud voice, 'Lazarus, come out!'"

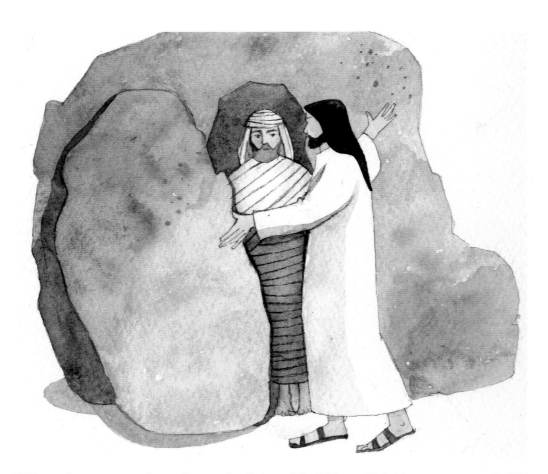

What happened to Jesus's friend? Why did Jesus weep? What miracle did Jesus perform?

I Remember

THE STORY OF THE HEALING OF THE BLIND MAN

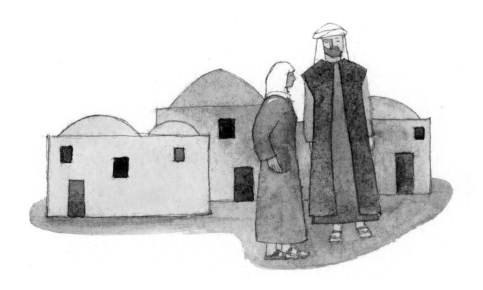

When Jesus touched the blind man's eyes,

his vision was restored.

"I can see clearly," he said with a shout,

then knelt before the Lord.

Mark 8:25-"Once more Jesus put his hands on the man's eyes. Then his eyes were opened, his sight was restored, and he saw everything clearly."

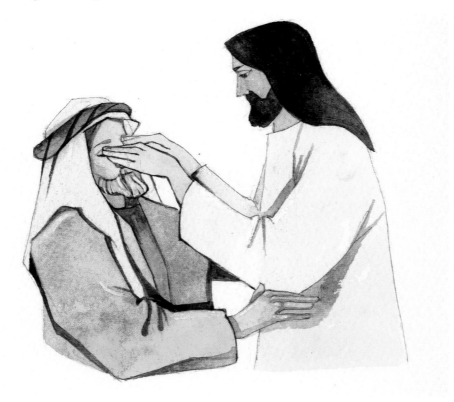

What was wrong with the man? How long had he been blind? What did Jesus do? Was the man able to see? How did he thank Jesus?

I Remember
THE RESURRECTION STORY

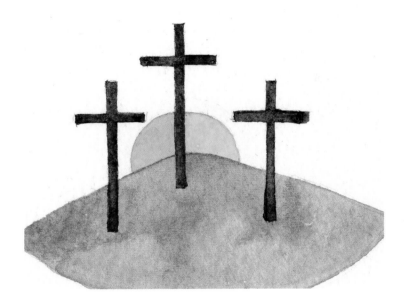

It was to save us from our sins that the cross he chose.

On the third day angels proclaimed, "Jesus Christ arose!"

Matthew 28: 5,6- "The angel said to the women, 'Do not be afraid, for I know that you are looking for Jesus, who was crucified. He is not here; he has risen, just as he said. Come and see the place where he lay.'"

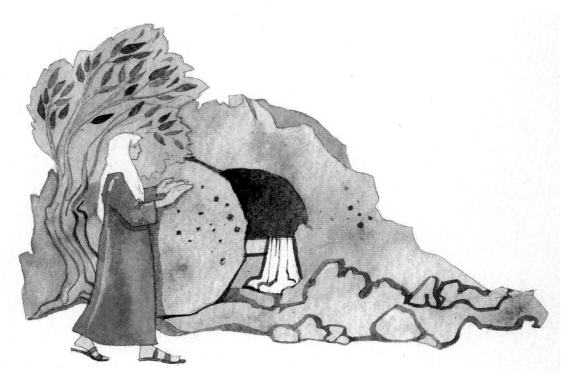

Who died on the cross? Why was he crucified? Where did they put his body? What happened on the third day? Why did the women go to the tomb? Who saw Jesus after that? Then where did Jesus go? Where is he, now?

"Jesus did many other things as well. If every one of them were written down, I suppose that even the whole world would not have room for the books that would be written."

John 21:25

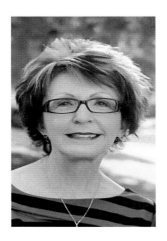

Brenda Poulos is a former elementary classroom teacher and counselor in Arizona. An avid reader and movie buff, she and her husband enjoy traveling, home remodeling and volunteering. Brenda is the best-selling author of *Runaways: The Long Journey Home, The Choice: Will's Last Testament, Simon Says,* and *I Remember the Seasons.*

Her mother's diagnosis of Alzheimer's in 2016 was the catalyst for the I REMEMBER series.

Find out more about the author on brendapoulos.org, spiritualsnippets.com, Facebook, Goodreads, and Twitter @mtnst14Brenda.

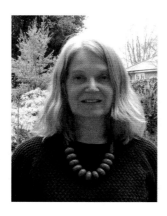

Jenny Reynish is an artist and illustrator who has created a wide variety of illustrations for US and UK publishers for children and adults. She has been drawing and painting for as long as she can remember and is always excited by the variety and surprises of new projects. Her individual style was sparked by a Persian rug which her aunt brought back from Isfahan. She loves the colours and decorative arts of India and the Middle East.

Jenny lives on the south coast of the UK in East Sussex and loves living by the sea in an area that provides ample inspiration for her work. She enjoys life drawing and printmaking, and is also an Iyengar Yoga teacher. She spent five years caring for her mother.

Her work can be seen at magiccarpetpics.co.uk , theaoi.com , and childrensillustrators.com.

ADDITIONAL ACTIVITIES FOR PEOPLE WITH ALZHEIMER'S

1. Recite Nursery Rhymes
2. Listen to music
3. Toss a ball
4. Blow bubbles
5. Sort and fold laundry
6. Color pictures
7. Clip coupons
8. Garden
9. Sort objects by shape/color
10. Rake leaves
11. Look at family photos
12. String beads
13. Sweep a patio, porch, or sidewalk
14. Do puzzles
15. Play board games
16. Work with clay
17. Paint pictures; finger paint
18. Fill a birdfeeder
19. Make a scrapbook
20. Wash windows
21. Sort coins, buttons, etc.
22. Roll yarn into a ball
23. Dance to favorite music
24. Play a musical instrument
25. Read picture books
26. Visit the zoo

Suggested Websites

www.alz.org

www.alzfdn.org

www.best-alzheimers-products.com/games-for-people-with-alzheimers.html

www.caring.com/articles/activities-for-dementia-alzheimers

Current Research/Statistics

www.alz.org/research

www.alzheimers.net/resources-alzheimers-statistics

www.mayoclinic.org/diseases-conditions/alzheimers-disease/in-depth/

Facebook

Please visit A.I.D. (Assisting Individuals with Dementia) where caregivers and interested people encourage others by sharing their knowledge, and stories with others.

Synopses of Bible Stories

Story 1- The Creation Story (Genesis 1:1-2:3)

God spoke in the darkness: "Let there be light!" And right away the darkness scattered. "From now on, when it's dark it will be 'night' and when it's light, it will be 'day'," God said.

On the second day, God made the earth and sky. On the third day, He put all the water in one place and all the dry land in another. God made plants and trees. On the fourth day, God made the sun, moon, and stars. The next day, God created millions of fish in the oceans. He made birds, too. And that was the end of the fifth day. On the sixth day, God added creatures to the land. He added Mankind to enjoy and take care of all that He had created.

After six days, the whole universe was completed. On the seventh day God rested.

Story 2- Adam and Eve (Genesis 2:8-3:24)

God took some clay and breathed into it and it became a living man who He called Adam.

The Lord made a garden for him to live in called Eden. It had streams of water, beautiful trees, and animals. Then He took a rib from Adam's side and made a woman. God told them, "All this is for you. Help yourself to anything, but never touch the tree in the middle of the Garden. It gives knowledge of good and evil. The day you eat its fruit, you will die."

One day, Eve was gathering berries for dinner when a snake urged her to eat its forbidden fruit.

"God has told us we cannot eat from The Tree of Good and Evil," Eve told the serpent.

The serpent lied. "God knows that if you eat from it you'll become just like God, and will be able to decide for yourself what is right and what is wrong."

The woman thought how delicious it looked and how good it would be to be wise and powerful like God. She ate the fruit and also gave some to Adam.

When they blamed each other for their sins, God told them that they had to leave the Garden of Eden, "From now on you'll have to make clothes and grow food. Nothing will come easily—not even childbirth. And one day, you will die."

Story 3- Baby Moses (Exodus 1:22-2:10)

A man and a woman from the tribe of Levi got married. She became pregnant and had a son by him. She saw that her baby was a fine child.

She hid him for three months because King Pharaoh had ordered that all male babies were to die. When she couldn't hide him any longer, she placed the child in a basket coated with tar and put it in the grass that grew along the bank of the Nile River.

When Pharaoh's daughter was bathing in the river, she saw the basket and sent her female slave to get it. When she opened it, she saw the baby. He was crying. "This is one of the Hebrew babies," she said.

Then the baby's sister walked up to her and asked, "Do you want me to go and get one of the Hebrew women? She could nurse the baby for you."

"Yes. Go," she answered. So the girl went and got the baby's mother.

Pharaoh's daughter told her, "Nurse this baby for me." So the woman took the baby and nursed him. When the child grew older, she took him to Pharaoh's daughter and he became her son. She named him Moses. She said, "I pulled him out of the water."

Story 4- David and Goliath (I Samuel 17:1-58)

In the midst of a battle between the Philistines and the Israelites, a shepherd boy named David was sent to the battlefield with provisions. When he arrived, he found that the soldiers were contemplating who might fight the Philistine giant, Goliath. "In keeping my father's sheep safe, I have killed both lions and bears. I will kill the giant for he has defied the armies of the living God."

He took a stone from his bag and put it into a sling and slung it, striking the Philistine Giant in the forehead. Then he drew a sword from its sheath and killed him.

Story 5- Daniel and the Lions' Den (Daniel 6:1-28)

When the Babylonians conquered Israel, one of the young men taken captive was Daniel.

Over the next several decades, Daniel led a life of hard work and obedience to God. Some government workers tricked King Darius into passing a decree that during a thirty-day period, anyone who prayed to another god or man besides the king would be thrown into the lions' den.

But, Daniel didn't change his habit of praying to God. When he was caught, King Darius was told. He wanted to revoke the decree, but he could not.

At sundown, Daniel was thrown into the den of lions. All night, the king worried about Daniel. Finally, at dawn, he ran to the lions' den and asked Daniel if his God had protected him.

Daniel replied, "My God sent his angel, and he shut the mouths of the lions. They haven't hurt me because I was found innocent in his sight. Nor have I ever done any wrong before you, O king."

The king issued another decree, ordering the people to worship the God of Daniel.

Story 6- Jonah and the Whale (Jonah 1-4)

God commanded Jonah to preach repentance to the city of Nineveh, a wicked city and one of Israel's fiercest enemies. However, Jonah ran away to the city of Tarshish.

On the voyage there, a violent storm threatened to break the ship apart. The terrified crew cast lots, determining that Jonah was responsible for the storm. Jonah told them to throw him overboard and when they did, the waters immediately grew calm.

Jonah was swallowed by a great fish, which God provided. Jonah was in the giant fish three days. When he repented, God commanded the whale, and it vomited him onto dry land. This time Jonah obeyed God, proclaiming to Nineveh that in forty days the city would be destroyed.

They believed Jonah's message and repented. God had compassion on them and did not destroy them.

Story 7- Noah and the Ark (Genesis 6:9-14)

God saw great wickedness on the earth and decided to destroy mankind. However, one righteous man named Noah found favor in God's eyes. So, God told Noah to build an ark for him and his family to save them from a flood He was going to send to destroy every living thing.

God also instructed Noah to bring into the ark two of all living creatures, both male and female, and seven pairs of all the clean animals, along with food for the animals and Noah's family.

After they entered the ark, rain fell on the earth for forty days and nights. The waters flooded the earth for a hundred and fifty days, and every living thing on the face of the earth was wiped out. As the waters receded, Noah and his family waited for the surface of the earth to dry out.

When they came out of the ark, Noah built an altar and worshiped the Lord. He promised never again to destroy all the living creatures with a flood. As a sign, God set a rainbow in the sky.

Story 8- The Birth of Jesus (Matthew 1-2; Luke 1-2)

Almost 2,000 years ago a young woman, named Mary was told by an angel that she would have a son named Jesus and that he would be the Son of God.

At this time, Mary was engaged to Joseph. The angel told Joseph that Mary would be pregnant from the Lord and she would have a son, Jesus, who would save the people from their sins.

Mary and Joseph had to sojourn to Bethlehem for the census. They arrived there after traveling for several days. However, they were told that the inns were full. Seeing that Mary was due to give birth at any moment, the owner of an inn told Joseph that they could stay in his stable. And, that is where Jesus was born. The only place for the baby to sleep was a manger.

An angel told shepherds the good news of the birth of the Savior and Messiah, Jesus Christ. They went immediately to find baby Jesus.

After some time, three wise men saw a brilliant star in the sky that rested over the stable. They, too, traveled to see Him, giving him gifts of gold, frankincense and myrrh.

Today we celebrate the birth of Jesus, our Savior, at Christmas time.

Story 9- Loaves and Fishes (Matthew 14:13-21)

One day, Jesus took the apostles into the desert to teach them privately. However, people started to follow them, hoping Jesus would heal the sick and teach them about the kingdom of God.

When it was getting late, Jesus told the apostles to give the people food. When they told Jesus the only food they had was that of a boy with five loaves of bread and two fishes, Jesus blessed the food. It was broken into pieces and passed out to all the people.

Everyone ate and was blessed. The apostles collected twelve baskets of leftovers!

Story 10- Lazarus (John 11:1-45)

When Lazarus fell ill, his sisters, Mary and Martha, sent a message to Jesus. Two days later, Jesus arrived at their home. By then, their brother had already been in the tomb four days.

"Lord," Mary said, "if you had been here, my brother would not have died." But he said, "Your brother will rise again."

Then Jesus said these important words: "I am the **resurrection** and the life. He who believes in me will live, even though he dies; and whoever lives and believes in me will never die."

Jesus wept with them. Then He prayed to God, and said, "Lazarus, come out!"

When he came out, many people put their faith in Jesus as a result of this incredible miracle.

Story 11- Jesus Heals the Blind Man (John 9:1-12)

One day Jesus and His disciples came across a man who had been born blind. He was begging for money.

Jesus' disciples asked Him, "Rabbi, was this man born blind because he sinned? Or did his parents sin?"

Jesus said, "This happened so that God's work could be shown in his life." Then, he spit on the ground and made some mud in his hands and put it on the man's eyes.

"Go," He told him. "Wash in the Pool of Siloam." So the man went and washed. And he came home able to see for the first time in his life! He told his neighbors what Jesus had done.

Story 12-The Resurrection

(Matthew 28:1-20; Mark 16:1-20; Luke 24:1-49; John 20:1-25)

After Jesus was crucified on the cross, his body was placed in a tomb and a large stone rolled to cover the entrance. Soldiers guarded the sealed tomb.

On the third day, a Sunday, several women went to the tomb at dawn to anoint his body.

A violent earthquake took place and an angel ro
Jesus was no longer there. Then he instructed t]
themselves.

The women ran to tell the disciples that Jesus had risen. But, Jesus met them on their way. They fell at his feet and worshiped him.

He said, "Do not be afraid. Go tell my brothers to go to Galilee. There they will see me."

When the guards reported what had happened to the chief priests, they bribed the soldiers to lie and say that the disciples had stolen the body in the night.

After his resurrection, Jesus visited the disciples while they were gathered at a house in prayer. He also talked to two of them on the road and others who were fishing at the Sea of Galilee.

Book was assembled Backwards. Start at other End (page 12) for Stories - Other Copy is Correct